# Who the Hell Are You?
## Alzheimer's the Wrong Diagnosis

### By Virginia Wright

Author Web: http://www.virginiawright.com
Email: info@virginiawright.com

CreateSpace Independent Publishing Platform
North Charleston, SC

First Edition 2017

Editor: Ingrid Hall
http://www.luv2write.net

ISBN-13: 978-1517224745
ISBN-10: 1517224748
LCCN: 2015917106

More books by this author available online:
http://www.amazon.com/author/virginiawright
http://www.barnesandnoble.com
http://www.booksamillion.com

## Dedication

To my beautiful mother, my best friend, my confidant, and my biggest cheerleader—R.I.P.

## Acknowledgement

David Wright, my husband, and my strength.

To my best friend, Kim Vorodi, many thanks for getting me through such a difficult time in my life.

Dennis Higgins, my virtual brother, and author buddy, for offering to read an advance copy of this book.

Deanie Dunne, author, and friend, for being my Beta reader.

Launa McNeilly, author, adopted sister, and friend, thank you for waiting.

# Who the Hell Are You?
# Alzheimer's the Wrong Diagnosis

## Prologue

For some time, my mother was not herself and initially diagnosed with Alzheimer's. The medications given to treat this condition did not help. And by the time a second opinion brought news with what was wrong, it was too late to save her. Tragically, she died.

I hope by telling this true story, "Who the Hell Are You: Alzheimer's the Wrong Diagnosis," it will help people identify symptoms of a condition that is similar to Alzheimer's, but, unlike Alzheimer's, if found in time—is treatable with a good outcome.

## *March 19, 2005*

I love birthday celebrations. Today's birthday would be no exception. The day started with phone calls bringing birthday wishes, birthday songs, and plans for my birthday dinner and all the usual birthday fanfare. One of my birthday calls was from my BFF, Kim. She is usually one of the first to call and wish me a happy birthday every year. Kim and I met when we were young girls, teenagers; as our husbands worked together overseas. When we left Europe, we kept in touch; it had been thirty plus years already, and we were like sisters. And why wouldn't I be excited by her birthday call? My excitement level that morning was lacking, as I was feeling a bit let down. The childish side of me was raising its ugly head because I had not received a call from another person that I held dear in my life, my mother. And *she was always the one* who made a big fuss over my birthday. Even though many miles separated us, Mum would get in touch with my husband or children, and send them money to buy me a cake, ice cream, balloons, and every year she made the celebration a little different.

Kim knew how hurt I was; she also knew that I was extremely concerned. Concerned because this was not like my mother to have missed my birthday, we both knew it. Even *you* will be able to tell that this was strange behavior on her part, just by what I have said about how she usually celebrated my birthday. I knew in my heart, she would never, ever, forget my birthday. I did not care about the gift, the cake, balloons, or money in a card. I just wanted to hear "Happy Birthday, my darling," from my mother. Growing up, she referred to me as her *little* darling. So hearing those particular words would have helped this forgotten day.

On TV, in the newspaper, and on the Internet, I had heard similar stories about situations like this, always told in a slightly different way. Repeatedly, the reports are about a parent forgetting special occasions, forgetting to take medications, or wandering off—calling it *Alzheimer's*.

Kim was friends with my mother, so she called and gently reminded her it was my birthday. When Mum finally called me, she exploded and told me she *had not* forgotten my birthday; she had planned to call late in the day in case I had gone out for supper.

This sounds plausible, right? But she never addressed the fact that she had not sent me anything for my birthday, not even a card; I never addressed that with her either.

After that day, life as I knew it changed with my mother, forever. The conversations got more and more bizarre as time went on. Subject matters became very different every time we spoke. Having Mum remember me, was vital. I didn't want her to forget her daughter. I copied some photos on my computer and printed them out to make a collage on paper; I sent these to Mum. I gave it time for mail to reach her; then I called to see what she would say; if she would remember me. Sadly, she didn't and instead said, "Who is that woman in the pictures you sent me?"

Over the next couple of years, Mum and I had lots of conversations on the phone. Even though she didn't recognize my face in the photographs, she did recognize my voice when I called her.

So the day my mother first started talking gibberish to me on the phone, I wondered whether she had recently had a stroke and might be suffering side effects from it—and I knew at that moment, things had gone from bad to worse.

First, I spoke with my stepfather about her behavior; he told me my mother had been acting out of the ordinary, peculiar, for quite some time. I strongly suggested he take her to the doctor. He asked if I would call her doctor first, and speak with him for any suggestions as to what could be wrong.

Because of the patient privacy laws, I understood what I was up against before I even called the doctor's office. But I was desperate for answers and felt it was worth a try.

I rang up the doctor and told him what was going on and asked if he could give me his best-educated guess as to what was wrong with my mother. He said, "Unfortunately, Virginia, it sounds like she has Alzheimer's." "I will have my nurse call her tomorrow, to set up an appointment where I can check her out."

But he informed me he could not give me more information about my mother due to the privacy laws.

My stepfather made sure Mum went to her doctor's appointment as scheduled. The doctor gave her a *diagnosis of and prescription for* Alzheimer's, to help ease her symptoms. But eventually, he also set her up for some medical testing.

**As time went on; my mother's memory increasingly diminished.**

Mum eventually forgot how to drive a car, and to do simple tasks like combing her hair, applying her makeup, making a bed and putting on her jeans. Walking seemed more like a chore, as if her feet were hard to pick up, so she shuffled when she walked. Her personality changed, she became angry easily and at times became violent.

My stepfather ten years her elder, said he could no longer handle her care alone. He put her on a list at a local nursing home, but they told him they had lots of people ahead of her. It could be a two-year wait.

My mother's care escalated, folks were coming in to clean the house that she had always kept immaculately. Other people were hired to sit with her while my stepfather tended to grocery shopping, financial affairs, and essential errands. Living out of state, I would get many calls over the next months as my stepfather found it increasingly difficult to deal with her behaviors. He wanted help, and he asked it of me.

Eventually, he moved my mother and all her lifelong possessions, lock, stock, and barrel to Ohio, to live next door to my husband and me. The plan was that I would help with the caring of Mum, and I did, for a short time.

I established a daily routine, which included making sure she had breakfast, and that she took her daily medications; then I would help her shower and get dressed.

Every day when I would go into the house, I would go over and kiss her on the cheek. I would usually say, "Mum, I am here to help you get ready for the day." But this particular morning when I arrived to check on her,  she startled me with her tone of voice as she said, *"Who the Hell Are You?"* My heart was crushed, torn—*no, broken.* My mother didn't know who I was. After I had taken a second or two to gather my feelings, I told her that it was her daughter, to close her eyes and listen to my voice, that it was her little darling. She didn't have a good day that day, and days that followed just seemed to get worse.

On my birthday that same year, March 19, 2007, I was able to celebrate with my mother one last time. It was the first time we had celebrated together in many years. We would have a pizza party with cake and ice cream. A joyful day, the old birthday hoorah! We carried the food in the house; we ate, and when it came to the lighting of the candles on my cake, my mother said, "Oh, good, it's *my* birthday, and we are celebrating."

She was so happy, and none of us in the room said a word otherwise about the fact that it was not her day to celebrate. Everyone sang happy birthday, but it was not to me, it was to Sheila, my mother.

Had I been lying to myself about how bad she was? Maybe. As I thought—maybe if I fed her well, eventually she would get better.

She had not been in the state of Ohio more than a couple of weeks when one of my daily checks entailed a crisis. My mother told me her stomach hurt. I took her to the bathroom and after she had finished, as she was getting up off the toilet; I saw blood in the bowl. Immediately, I called my stepfather and husband in to see what I saw. We wasted no time, we put my mother in the car and took her to the nearest emergency room.

After the docs had examined her, they had her give them a urine sample in a cup and sent it off to the lab. It turns out; she had a urinary tract infection (UTI), and that explained the blood earlier at home. But, they took me aside and said that they were concerned over how bizarre my mother was acting.

I said matter of factly that she had Alzheimer's. I only regurgitated what her doctor back home had told me. But, these doctors wanted to do a computerized tomography (CT) scan straight away, to look at her brain. We agreed that would be a good idea, under the circumstances.

## *Diagnosis*

A couple of hours after testing, a neurologist came back and asked if we would step into his office as he wanted to show us her brain scan and go over the results. He began explaining that my mother, more than likely, *would not* have benefitted from taking the Alzheimer's medication prescribed and had been on for the last two plus years. He continued to explain that she had a condition called "Hydrocephalus." Hydro what, I thought, and then asked, "What's that?" He began to tell us that *hydrocephalus is a condition in which excess cerebrospinal fluid (CSF) abnormally builds up in the ventricles of the brain.* And the fluid may cause increased pressure in the head.

However, what my mother had he said, was *normal pressure* hydrocephalus (NPH). Then he went on to say, that in some instances of NPH, the Alzheimer's type *symptoms can reverse* with a surgical procedure such as by shunt placement in the brain, and *with a good outcome!*

## Prognosis

The neurologist asked for us to have my mother's last two years of medical records faxed to them and any CT scans that she may have had done. Thankfully, the hospital in Maine got right back to the Ohio hospital. After reviewing my mother's records, the doctor said that the prognosis of hydrocephalus depended on the extent of her symptoms; and the delay in diagnosis and treatment she had or didn't have.

*Some people are born with hydrocephalus; NPH may take place from an illness or a fall with a head injury. While Hydrocephalus is a chronic condition, with early diagnosis and appropriate treatment— (i.e., surgery and medical equipment such as a brain shunt), many people can lead a near normal life.*

Originally, in my mother's case, as mentioned earlier, her initial diagnosis was Alzheimer's. While her symptoms of dementia were similar to this condition, she also had a telltale sign of NPH, with her unusual gait. She walked as if her feet were weighted down.

When the neurologist in Ohio told us my mother had NPH, he said that not only did her current CT scan show this, but the one faxed to him from two years earlier did, too. We do not know how long she had been living with NPH, but looking back, we assume for at least two years based on the symptoms she had been having. We also think a fall on the ice with a head injury a few years earlier, while walking her dog, may have caused this.

The Ohio neurologist set up an appointment for my mother to visit a neurosurgeon in Pittsburgh, Pennsylvania.

An ambulance took her to the clinic, where she had an examination. We were ecstatic as the doctor said her heart sounded good, all other vitals were well enough to make her a good candidate to do a *brain shunt surgery*. After shunt placement, the doctor said that she would see the neurosurgeon within a month for a check-up and possible brain shunt adjustment.

## *I Love You*

I must have said, "I love you" three hundred times during my mother's hospital stay. Just as many times, I must have told her what a good mother she was. And, I talked to her endlessly about things I remembered as a child growing up in hopes to jog her memory. In the past, she often spoke fondly of her Grampy Dutch, whom she adored. There were times that through that empty gaze, she would look up towards the corner of the room as if she could see him, and she would call out the word, Grampy.

They placed the brain shunt; we were thrilled, *actually hopeful.* However, in the process of not being well and staying in bed for several weeks, Mum had developed blood clots. Mum went into surgery to try and catch the clots and hopefully to prevent them from reaching her lungs. After a successful surgery, she came down with double pneumonia and urosepsis from her UTI.

*Mum eventually completely forgot the faces of people she loved, her husband, children, grandchildren, and yes, me, her little darling.*

## The Kiss of Death
### May 31st, 2007

Mum died peacefully; she took one last deep breath, and she was gone. I can honestly say, that in my entire life, I have never sobbed as much as I did that day. My heart felt as if it was breaking in two.

Thoughts began filling my head, such as if her doctor had not given her an initial diagnosis of Alzheimer's, perhaps she would have been enjoying her life with us on that day. She could have had extra time to spend with her children, grandchildren, great-grandchildren, and time to enjoy warm summer rains, time to marvel at the sight of a rainbow, and time to spend with...*me*.

## *Gratefulness*

Yes, gratefulness. Gratefulness because I had those last few days with my mother. Even with it being a horrific time—and with my heart breaking to see her dying; at the same time, I felt privileged to be with her in a private moment such as death.

I was comforted being by her side—stroking her hair, holding her hand, telling her stories from the past and praying for her on the way out of her earthly life.

These gestures of mine were so fitting, right even, since in the past she had so lovingly held my hand, stroked my hair when I was sick, told me stories and prayed our nighttime prayers, night after night when I was a little girl.

Losing my mother to the wrong diagnosis was such a painful time in my life. Writing about it helped me work through a difficult period, which some may say was the only reason I told her story.

But in truth, while this is partly the reason, it is not the main reason; writing this story was to help others recognize a condition normal pressure hydrocephalus, as opposed to Alzheimer's. I implore you to ask questions of your doctors and get second opinions if you have doubts about an Alzheimer's diagnosis. It is *your* right, *your loved one's* right.

Do not let your mother, grandmother, aunt, sister, brother, father, uncle, husband, cousin— loved ones, slip through the fingers of the medical chaos. The correct diagnosis of a family member could mean the difference between living a full earthly lifespan, or not.

## Conclusion

Please take from this accounting of my mother's death one thing—and that is, not to be afraid to ask for a second opinion from a doctor. Do not be afraid to question a diagnosis. Be proactive, if you have Internet access do research from several reputable sources, to look at all of the options available.

If you live away from a parent, and they are sick, they can't always help themselves. Seek a trusted neighbor or another third party as an advocate for your loved one.

When both parents are elderly, go with or get someone to go to the doctor appointments with them if you cannot. Being the third ear can help with decisions that may not be made well necessarily by the elderly when they are sick or confused. Most major hospitals have counselors or patient liaisons to assist families. Ask for a medical contact at the hospital if necessary.

My stepfather did not have a patient advocate helping him. I never had another conversation with Mum's doctor. However, he did have further medical testing done as he mentioned he would, on her visit. I say the initial diagnosis of Alzheimer's was the beginning of a series of mishaps for Mum that sealed her fate, but I hold no malice against her physician. That testing he talked about doing showed as my stepfather put it, *a spot on her brain.*

That spot we learned later from the Ohio doctors was the enlarged ventricles, the NPH, showing up on the scan. The first team of specialists knew Mum had this condition, and they suggested a brain shunt placement out of state, as they could not do it in Maine. My stepfather, being elderly, we don't believe understood this, or what it all meant for my mother if she didn't have it. A patient liaison would have been helpful in this case.

My mother lived the last months of her life with horrible migraine headaches. She continued to deteriorate needlessly.

*Advocate for your loved ones, ask questions, research, get second opinions—get someone to listen to symptoms.*

If after reading about my mother's accounting of normal pressure hydrocephalus or from searching the sources listed, you have an "aha moment," talk to your loved one's doctor. If insurance allows, seek appropriate testing from a specialist who can treat brain conditions— to give you a prompt and proper diagnosis.

*Symptoms of Normal Pressure Hydrocephalus*

- **Difficulty walking, (unusual Gait) as if the feet are weighted down or glued to the floor, with shuffling.**
- **Forgetfulness**
- **Incontinence, (Bladder problems)**

These are two digitally drawn brain images, one with NPH, and enlarged ventricles and the other brain image is with the normal ventricles.

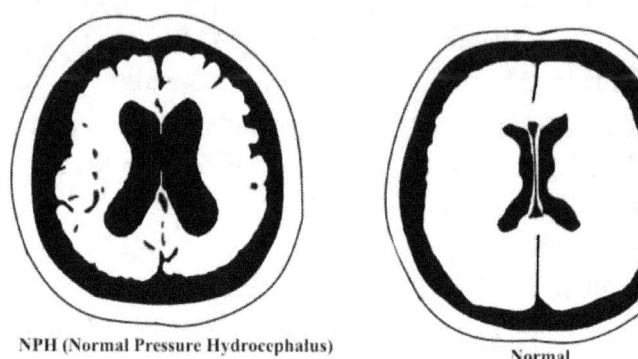

NPH (Normal Pressure Hydrocephalus)

Normal

*The images are not meant to be an accurate drawing of the brain, rather, a rough idea of what NPH looks like compared to standard.

*Normal Pressure Hydrocephalus, in many cases, will go unrecognized and misdiagnosed as Alzheimer's as they have similar symptoms.*

### *What is Normal Pressure Hydrocephalus (NPH)?*

The ventricles in the brain enlarge with NPH but with no or little pressure. However, despite the name *normal pressure* hydrocephalus, cerebrospinal fluid (CSF) pressures can fluctuate.

### *NPH Treatments*

Shunt placement, to keep intracranial pressure within reasonable limits by diverting the CSF away from the brain is one possible treatment; this is the surgery my mother eventually had. An alternative treatment would be surgery whereby a tiny hole made in the third ventricle, called endoscopic third ventriculostomy, is made and creates a new path for CSF to flow.

***Treated Normal Pressure Hydrocephalus can have a good prognosis if dealt with promptly.***

My hope with this story is that you find it enlightening, and a tad educational. Hopefully, you never have the misdiagnosis tragedy in your family that we have endured in ours.

*-Virginia Wright*

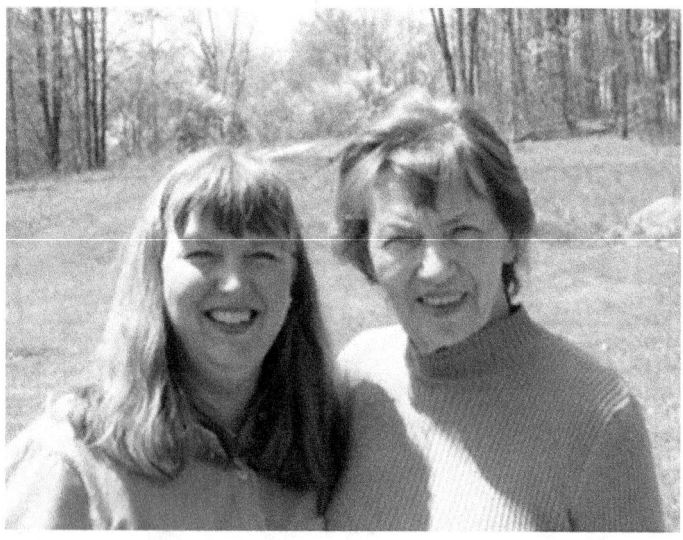

*This photo is one year before my mother died. At the time, we thought she had Alzheimer's. Sadly, while initially diagnosed and treated for that condition, it was the wrong diagnosis. Mum, (right), had NPH.*

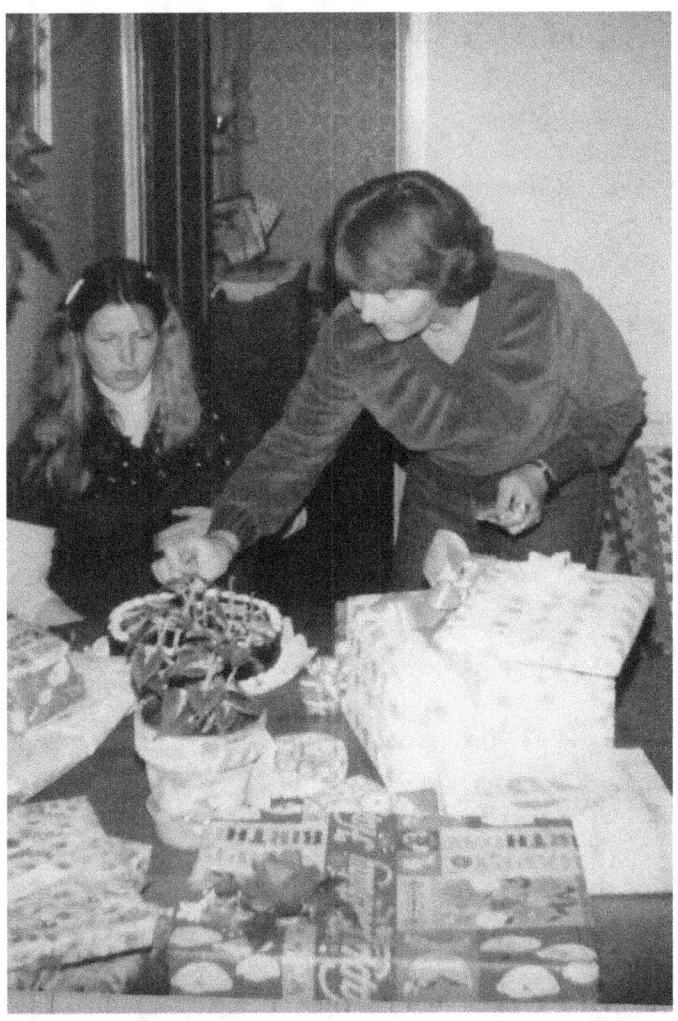

*March 1981, Mum before NPH, lighting candles on my birthday cake. If you look close, you can see a smile on her face. She loved making my birthday special!*

## *Additional Information & Sources*

*The websites listed offer information about various types of hydrocephalus, Alzheimer's, support services and more.*

**National Hydrocephalus Foundation**

Hydrocephalus Association
4340 East West Highway
Suite 905
Bethesda, MD 20814-4447
Telephone: 301-202-3811 / 888-598-3789
Fax: 301-202-3813
Email: info@hydroassoc.org

**Hydrocephalus-Association**

http://www.hydroassoc.org/

**\*\*September is Hydrocephalus Awareness Month**  http://www.hydroassoc.org/september-is-hydrocephalus-awareness-month-heres-what-you-can-do/

**What is Normal Pressure Hydrocephalus?**

http://www.hydroassoc.org/normal-pressure-hydrocephalus

## Research – Division of Neuroscience

*http://www.nia.nih.gov/research/dn*

## Alzheimer's Foundation of America

http://www.alzfdn.org
*For more information, contact the Alzheimer's Foundation of America. Call 866.232.8484.*

## Alzfdn Twitter

*https://twitter.com/alzfdn*

## Alzheimer's Association

*https://www.alz.org/*
*24/7 Helpline: 1.800.272.3900*

## Alzheimer's Association Twitter
*https://twitter.com/alzassociation*

## Long-Distance Caregiving

http://www.nia.nih.gov/health/publication/so-far-away-twenty-questions-and-answers-about-long-distance-caregiving

### American Health Care Association (AHCA):

The nation's largest association of long term and post-acute care providers. http://www.ahcancal.org

### National Long-Term Care Ombudsman Resource Center:

http://www.ltcombudsman.org/ombudsman

### Talking With Your Doctor:
### National Institute on Aging

http://www.nia.nih.gov/health/publication/talking-your-doctor-presentation-toolkit?utm_source=health-aging&utm_medium=website&utm_content=TWY DPT&utm_campaign=HA_Featured

### American Society on Aging
*http://www.asaging.org/*

### Twitter:
*https://twitter.com/ASAging*

## Notes:

## Notes: